I0427977

Cleansetox

Lose 20 pounds in 10 days!

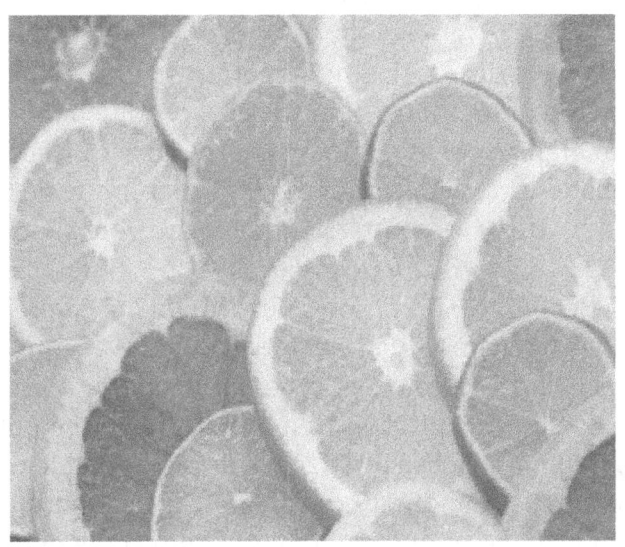

Cristie Will

Cleansetox
Lose 20 pounds in 10 days!
Copyright © 2015 by Cristie Will

All rights reserved. No part of this book may be reproduced in any form or by any electronic or mechanical means, including information storage and retrieval systems, without permission in writing from the author. For information, contact Cristie Will at cristiewill@outlook.com.

The content of this book is for general instruction only. Each person's physical, emotional, and spiritual condition is unique. The instruction in this book is not intended to replace or interrupt the reader's relationship with a physician or other professional. Please consult your doctor for matters pertaining to your specific health and diet.

All rights reserved. No part of this publication may be reproduced, distributed, or transmitted in any form or by any means, including photocopying, recording, or other electronic or mechanical methods, without the prior written permission of the publisher or author, except in the case of brief quotations embodied in critical reviews and certain other noncommercial uses permitted by copyright law. For permission requests, email the publisher or author at cristiewill@outlook.com or send your request to 336 Ricker Lane, Johnstown, CO 80534.

To contact the publisher and or Author, visit www.cbwill.com or www.healthtidings.com
ISBN-13:9781511856119
ISBN-10:1511856114
Printed in the United States of America

Dedication

I want to dedicate this book to Maryellen Madden, my amazing friend that has helped so much. God Bless Maryellen!

Cleansetox
Lose 20 pounds in 10 days!

Acknowledgements

I want to thank Maryellen for introducing me to the Master Cleanser by Stanley Burroughs seven years ago. Cleansing is one of the most important things we can do for our mind, body and spirit and I gained that knowledge from Maryellen.

I also want to thank my daughter Lauren for her continued support and help when I need it.

I want to thank my brother Randy for all his help and ideas as well.

Introduction

I have evolved and transformed over the last seven years and hope to help others do the same.

Cleansetox is the stepping stone to gain your health back or to strengthen your health if you are already fairly healthy.

Cleansetox is a great stepping stone to weight loss. The saying is true "it takes three weeks to make or break a habit". By following the Cleansetox this will propel your weight loss and get you started in the right direction of your transformation.

 I have done just about all the popular cleanses plus figuring out this one. I took some classes and obtained my certification in Cleansing/Detoxing. This has helped me to understand even more.

Cleansetox has evolved through my introduction to the Master Cleanse, to my own trials and errors to my education in cleansing.

I want to share what I have done, what I know and what works for me. The Cleansetox is tried and true fore it can work for you too.

Keep in mind we are all different and to ALWAYS listen to your body. You are the one living in your body and you know.

Here's to good health and weight loss!

Cristie

Chapter 1
Cleansetox

Why Cleansing/Detoxing? Cleansing/Detoxing is the stepping stone to the elimination of every disease. As different health gurus have said "cure one disease you cure them all".

Stanley Burroughs says "As we eliminate and correct one disease, we correct them all, for every disease is corrected by the same process of cleansing and building positive good health."

My whole body, mind and spirit was deathly ill and toxic. I had to find a solution and quick. The Master Cleanse does work, but I just found it a bit harder, so I kept at it until I founded Cleansetox.

With all the highly processed things we eat and our high fast paced lives it's no wonder we are so toxic. I say highly processed things because we are no longer eating food since all the nutrients are processed right out of the food.

Our bodies are unique amazing machines. We have been given the food to keep our bodies healthy and highly effective, but we grab too much junk on the go.

When we don't give our bodies the right nutrients then before long we start depleting our bodies of nutrients and the next thing you know problems start popping up. Once one problem pops up before long another then another.

Our bodies, mind and spirt are like a high end machine that has to be cleaned and maintained to keep it going. If not it breaks down and often times has to have new parts, or live in pain and lastly dying, often times too young.

We do not have to grow old and decrepit.   If you need more reinforcement just go to an old folk's home.   Next take a look at people that are well into their 90's living at home and still driving, gardening etc.

There is so much information out there that it's enough for a person to want to throw their hands up and say "What am I supposed to do"?

One thing for certain we as a society have made it harder and we need to get back to the basics of life, but until we do then Cleansetox to keep yourself as healthy as possible.

Cleansetox will always be a go to healing, maintenance and weight loss aid. Even when we start eating organic and healthy there are still thousands of toxins bombarding us daily, such as the toxins in the air we breathe, our beauty skin care products, colognes and cleaning products just to mention a few things. I will provide you with ideas, recipes and alternatives to help rid more toxins on a daily basis.

Once you read about what food coloring alone can do to disrupt our systems you will want to do your best to be cognizant of what you are breathing and put into your body. I will be getting into more of what food coloring and toxins are doing. I will just touch on the tip of the iceberg though, having said that it will be enough for you to think, act and do even more research on your own.

Have you noticed over the years ADD/ADHD, Autism, Diabetes, Cancer, Heart Problems, Obesity, Depression just to name a few illnesses have steadily gone up year after year? This is due to all the chemicals, toxins, preservatives, additives, food coloring, MSG, Sugar, especially high fructose corn syrup and other things I haven't mentioned.

Speaking of sugar did you know there are 57 names and counting of sugar?

57 Names of Sugar and Sugar Aliases

1. Agave Nectar
2. Barley Malt
3. Beet Sugar
4. Black Strap Molasses
5. Brown Rice Syrup
6. Brown Sugar
7. Buttered Sugar
8. Cane Juice Crystals
9. Cane Juice
10. Cane Sugar
11. Caramel
12. Carob Syrup
13. Caster Sugar
14. Coconut Sugar
15. Corn Sweetner
16. Corn Syrup
17. Corn Syrup Solids
18. Crystalline Frutose
19. Date Sugar
20. Demara Sugar
21. Dextran
22. Diastatic Malt
23. Diatase
24. Ethyl Maltol
25. Evaporated Cane Juice
26. Fructose
27. Fruit Juice Concentrates
28. Galactose
29. Glucose
30. Golden Sugar
31. Golden Syrup
32. High Fructose Corn Syrup
33. Honey
34. Invert Sugar
35. Lactose
36. Malt Syrup
37. Maltodextrin
38. Maltose
39. Maple Syrup
40. Molasses Syrup
41. Muscovado Sugar
42. Organic Raw Sugar
43. Oat Syrup
44. Panela
45. Panocha
46. Confectioner's Sugar
47. Rice Bran Syrup
48. Rice Syrup
49. Sorghum
50. Sorghum Syrup
51. Sucrose
52. Sugar
53. Syrup
54. Treacle
55. Tapioca Syrup
56. Turbinado Syrup
57. Yellow Sugar

Think again if you think you are not eating sugar.

MSG the silent deadly killer

MSG the common food additive now linked to weight gain according to an article I read. This is not at all surprising. I will list what names I can find on MSG for your convenience and list some of the symptoms as well. Here's a quote from the article and the link to it.

"In the latest research ... [scientists] followed more than 10,000 adults in China for about 5.5 years on average. The researchers measured MSG intake directly by before-and-after weighing of products, such as bottles of soy sauce, to see how much people ate ... Men and women who ate the most MSG (a median of 5 grams a day) were about 30 percent more likely to become overweight by the end of the study".

http://articles.mercola.com/sites/articles/archive/2011/06/16/this-common-food-additive-now-linked-to-weight-gain.aspx

MSG-induced brain lesions in the area of the hypothalamus and/or accumulations of glutamic acid have been shown to cause each of the following:

Retinal degeneration   Stunted Growth
Neuroendocrine disorders   Behavior Disorders
Obesity   Learning & Memory Disorders
Reproductive disorders   Hyperglycemia

In addition, there is a copious literature on addiction, stroke, epilepsy, degenerative disorders (Alzheimer's disease, Parkinson's disease, and ALS, for example), brain trauma, neuropathic pain, schizophrenia, anxiety, and depression, seemingly diverse disease processes of the central nervous system that appear to be associated with the "glutamate cascade." See link for more information. http://www.truthinlabeling.org/Dang.html

MSG Lists to be aware of:

Autolyzed Yeast
Glutamate
Monopotassium Glutamate
Monosodium Glutamate
Sodium Caseinate
Textured Protein
Calcium Caseinate
Glutamic Acid
Hydrolyzed Protein
Flavors and Flavorings
Natural Chicken Flavoring
Anything Enzyme Modified
Protease
Seasonings
Soy Sauce
Carrageenan
Corn Starch
Anything Ultra Pasteurized
Natural Flavors and Flavorings
Soy Protein Isolate
Malt Extract
Maltodextrin
Citric Acid
Natural Pork Flavoring
Soy Protein
Malt Flavoring
Powdered Milk
Natural Beef Flavoring
Barley Malt
Enzymes
Anything Protein Fortified

Yeast Extract
Yeast Food
Yeast Nutrient
Gelatin
Stock
Broth
Pectin
Bouillon

Remember this list can change anytime with manufacturers trying to hide toxic stuff. I don't believe they do it for harm they are in business and have to extend shelf life when can, but at the same time we don't need to buy their stuff.

Additives List

Here's a list of some of the most medically questionable and harmful additives in everyday foods:
1. Sodium nitrite
2. BHA & BHT
3. Propyl gallate
4. Monosodium glutamate
5. Trans fats
6. Aspartame
7. Acesulfame-K
8. Food colorings (Blue, Red, Green, Yellow)
9. Olestra
10. Potassium bromate
11. White sugar
12. Sodium chloride (salt)

Remember these list can and do change. These are most common and may appear in other lists I give you.

Toxic Food Dyes List

Here are some of the most common food dyes used today, according to the Food Freedom Network:

Blue #1 (Brilliant Blue) An unpublished study suggested the possibility that Blue 1 caused kidney tumors in mice. *What it's in:* Baked goods, beverages, desert powders, candies, cereal, drugs, and other products.

Blue #2 (Indigo Carmine) Causes a statistically significant incidence of tumors, particularly brain gliomas, in male rats. *What it's in:* Colored beverages, candies, pet food, & other food and drugs.

Toxic Food Dyes List Continued

Citrus Red #2 it's toxic to rodents at modest levels and caused tumors of the urinary bladder and possibly other organs. *What it's in:* Skins of Florida oranges.

Green #3 (Fast Green) Caused significant increases in bladder and testes tumors in male rats. *What it's in:* Drugs, personal care products, cosmetic products except in eye area, candies, beverages, ice cream, sorbet, ingested drugs, lipsticks, and externally applied cosmetics.

Red #3 (Erythrosine) Recognized in 1990 by the FDA as a thyroid carcinogen in animals and is banned in cosmetics and externally applied drugs. *What it's in:* Sausage casings, oral medication, maraschino cherries, baked goods, and candies.

Red #40 (Allura Red) This is the most-widely used and consumed dye. It may accelerate the appearance of immune system tumors in mice. It also causes hypersensitivity (allergy-like) reactions in some consumers and might trigger hyperactivity in children. *What it's in:* Beverages, bakery goods, dessert powders, candies, cereals, foods, drugs, and cosmetics.

Yellow #5 (Tartrazine) Yellow 5 causes sometimes-severe hypersensitivity reactions and might trigger hyperactivity and other behavioral effects in children. *What it's in:* Pet foods, numerous bakery goods, beverages, dessert powders, candies, cereals, gelatin desserts, and many other foods, as well as pharmaceuticals and cosmetics.

Yellow #6 (Sunset Yellow) Caused adrenal tumors in animals and occasionally causes severe hypersensitivity reactions. *What it's in:* Color bakery goods, cereals, beverages, dessert powders, candies, gelatin deserts, sausage, cosmetics, and drugs.

List of Corn Aliases

A surprising new food source may be causing you stomach irritation. Your body can be treating genetically modified corn sources as a toxin, which triggers a number of gastrointestinal issues. If you suspect that you may have a corn sensitivity, this list of possible corn sources can help you eliminate it from your diet.

Alpha tocopherol
Ascorbic acid
Baking powder
Calcium stearate
Caramel
Cellulose
Citric acid
Corn flour
Corn oil
Cornmeal
Cornstarch
Corn syrup
Dextrin
Dextrose (glucose)
Distilled white vinegar
Diglycerides
Ethylene
Ethyl acetate
Ethyl lactate
Fibersol-2
Fructose
Fumaric acid
Gluten (corn gluten)
Golden syrup
High fructose corn syrup
Inositol PolydextroseSorbitol

Polenta
PolydextroseSorbitol
Starch
Sucrose
Treacle
Vanilla extract
Xanthan gum
Xylitol
Zein
Invert Sugar
Malt
Maltodextrin
Margarine
Monoglycerides
Monosodium glutamate

List of Names for Dangerous Artificial Sweeteners

Ace K

Equal Spoonful

Sunett

APM

AminoSweet (but not in US)

Aspartyl-phenylalanine-1-methyl

Equal NatraTaste

Calcium cyclamate

Cologran = cyclamate and saccharin; not in US Sucaryl

Zerose ZSweet

Glycerin

Glycerine

Licorice

ClearCut Isomalt Decomalt

DiabetiSweet (also contains Acesulfame-K) Hydrogenated

Isomaltulose

Isomaltitol

Sugar alcohol

Maltitol Syrup Maltitol Powder

Hydrogenated High Maltose Content Glucose Syrup

Hydrogenated Maltose

Lesys

MaltiSweet (hard to find online to buy) SweetPearl

Acid saccharin Equal Saccharin Necta Sweet Sodium Saccharin

Sweet Twin

D-glucitol

D-glucitol syrup

Rebiana

1',4,6'-Trichlorogalactosucrose Trichlorosucrose

Equal Sucralose NatraTaste Gold

Natrulose

Xylipure Xylosweet

Sweet N Low

Sweet One

Smart Sweet

TwinSweet

NutraSweet

Splenda

Clean 15 and Dirty 15 Lists

Organic:	Non- organic:
Apples	Avocados
Strawberries	Sweet Corn
Grapes	Pineapples
Celery	Cabbage
Peaches	Sweet peas (frozen)
Spinach	Onions
Sweet bell peppers	Asparagus
Nectarines (imported)	Mangoes
Cucumbers	Papayas
Cherry tomatoes	Kiwi
Snap peas (imported)	Eggplant
Potatoes	Grapefruit
Hot peppers	Cantaloupe (domestic)
Blueberries (domestic)	Cauliflower
Zucchini	Sweet potatoes

Ok this is the main things to look out for in our foods. A good rule of thumb is if it has more than five items in an ingredients list it's probably not good to consume.

All these lists are a huge reason to Cleansetox about every 3 months or twice a year. Even if you don't consume any of these toxic chemicals you still are breathing them in and getting them other places, so Cleansetox is important. By cutting these out you are making a huge healthy change.

Chapter 2
Cleansetox Formula

I will get to the good part shortly, the Cleansetox Formula, but I want to share my cleansing detoxing experiences.

I started my first real cleanse in 2008 and I tried doing the Master Cleanse several times and I never made it the full ten days until I tried it again in 2012 and made it many times after that.

In 2012 I made it the full 10 days twice and then twice in 2013. I started out several other times and I just got to where I wouldn't make it the full 10 days. This is when I decided to do some homework and experiment with my findings. I also went back to school to obtain my certification in Cleansing.

What I found that is so important with any kind of Cleanse/Detoxing/Fast is you have to be able to stick it out.

1. You need a system you can go the distance with.
2. You need to make a commitment to do it. You need to be at least at an 8, between 1 and 10, 10 being the highest in order to stick it out.
3. You need to have your system prepared such as having what you need for the next ten days.
4. If you have family you live with and you're the mom/wife or the one in charge of the household duties then you need to plan ahead for them for 10 days. You want to set yourself up for success or don't do it until you are fully ready. For my family I would cook all weekend preparing things and freezing them so they could easily defrost, heat up and eat.
5. Mondays are always the best time to start a new change like a Cleanse or diet. Studies show by starting on a Monday the success rates are higher.

Once you do these five steps you are ready to transform.

Now getting to the good part. What is the Cleansetox Formula?
Let's go over the purpose, when and how to use the Cleansetox first
and then what to get.

Think of it as giving each and every cell, organ, and system in your
mind, body and spirit as a good shower, rinsing away all the toxic
waste.

Cleansetox is going to help break down toxins that have caused the
congestion in your body and mind. This will clean out your kidneys,
digestive system, glands, joints, muscles, nerves, arteries, blood
supply, blood vessels, and basically help keep you youthful each and
every day.

When you should Cleansetox is preferably every three months a year
or at the very least every six months, so twice a year. If in between
the times you Cleansetox and start to get really sick with chronic
issues like overweight starting to be a problem or maybe your
digestive system needs a break then Cleansetox at those times too.

Length of time is follow the Cleansetox for a minimum of 10 days or
more, but not more than 40 days at any one stretch. The Cleansetox
has all the nutrition needed during the time you are on it, providing
you are following what you are supposed to.

AS ALWAYS CONSULT YOUR PHYSICIAN BEFORE STARTING THIS OR
ANY DIET AND EXERCISE PLAN.

It's always best to use fresh organic produce when you can. If there
is a situation where you can't get fresh or its just way to
inconvenient then I found 100% pure organic juices in glass
containers and it's actually easier and cheaper. I have used the fresh
and this that I am going to tell you more about and I feel the same
on them.

You can get the "Italian Volcano 100% Organic Lemon Juice, Italian Volcano 100% Organic Lime Juice, and Italian Volcano 100% Organic Orange Juice. I have found the Lemon Juice at Costco and all 3 online. The Two bottles from Costco is approximately 80 lemons worth.

There will be naysayers say oh you can't drink the Lemon Juice even if it says its Organic, but you can just do Not Use ReaLemon it has preservatives. I haven't checked any other lemon juice since I found the Italian Volcano 100% Organic Juices.

You need to drink three 32 ounce drinks a day. I have a glass drinking glass with a straw that is 32 ounces and that is what I use.

Cleansetox Formula

Drink three 32 ounces a day equaling 96 ounces.

2 Tbsp	Lemon Juice
2 Tbsp	Lime Juice
2 Tbsp	Orange Juice
2 Tbsp	Maple Syrup, Grade B (has much more nutrients)
1/3 Tsp	Cayenne Pepper

Finish filling your container with filtered water.

Drink 96 ounces of this Formula each day for 10 days. Depending on your conditions you can go longer if you have checked with your physician and otherwise no problems. If you have been doing the Cleansetox for ten days you should have just an overwhelming sense of wellbeing. Other than just missing eating to socialize I could have gone on for much longer at a time. I have variations to the Cleansetox this is the straightforward way. I add the variations so that I have options to carry me to the finish line.

People ask why I add lime and orange juice. My answer is do make it more palatable and change it up, but get the great nutrients all at the same time.

Variations of the Cleansetox

Take the 6 tablespoons of lemon, lime and orange juice and mix it up. Sometimes I have 3 tablespoons of lemon, 3 tablespoons of orange and have changed it up other ways. I make sure I get some of each of the juices daily though. I have also had 6 tablespoons of orange juice leaving out the lemon and lime in my drink, but that's only once in a while.

There were times that I felt like I just couldn't do it and so I incorporated a little organic raw veggies. The Organic raw veggies have to be green is the biggest rule and of course nothing on them. The reason for Organic green only veggies is they have the highest nutritional content and lower in calories too. I only incorporate the raw veggies when I am having a difficult time with my Cleansetox and this will carry you to the finish line often times.

I always lose about the same no matter my variations. I lose anywhere between 18 to 22 pounds in 10 full days. I say ten full days because I will weigh myself in the morning on the 11th day of my Cleansetox. Yes I always weigh naked or in my underwear. You will also lose inches, so measure yourself to see even greater results.

Rest of the Cleansetox Formula is to drink one cup of tea at night to help you keep your colon flushed. The tea needs to be basically an herbal laxative tea like the Dieter's tea for example.

At the end of the Cleansetox you will need to slowly introduce food into your system whether its 10 days or more. You will find my soup recipes in the back to help you acclimate back into eating right. If you are wanting to keep your weight off or most of it that you lost then this is vital you stay at it to the very end.

The first couple of times I followed the Master Cleanse I would make it the 10 days and the 11th day I would dive off the deep end and eat bad and within a couple of weeks regain probably 12 of the 20 pounds back. I am telling you this so you understand what to do.

First day off of the Cleansetox you need to sip on just orange juice throughout the first day.

Second day off of the Cleansetox sip on orange juice and organic vegetable broth.

Third day off of the Cleansetox sip on orange juice, organic vegetable broth and soup (one of my recipes in the back).

Fourth day off of the Cleansetox eat all the soup all day you want, one of my recipes in the back.

Fifth day off of the Cleansetox resume eating normally. I would encourage you to eat 50% of your food intake for the day to be raw veggies and fruit to snack on, eat salads and find healthy dishes you can make for raw veggies.

At the end of ten days you will feel euphoric, so stay with it as long as you feel good. Remember to pay attention to your body and check with your doctor before going on any diet or exercise plan.

Be sure to read the chapter on frequently asked questions to answer any questions you may have.

What about Honey

Some say no Honey, but I say it's great to use if you can't handle the Maple Syrup and is a good equal to Maple Syrup. The studies show how effective and healthy Honey is. As you can see honey's nutrition facts has many of the same benefits. You can read much more about honey with the link I provided below the nutrition facts. Do you realize that honey is still good after 1,000's of years? It's one of the only things that doesn't spoil, so it's a safe bet in my book.

Minerals

Amounts Per Serving Size 339 g (1 Cup)		%DV
Calcium	20.3 mg	2%
Iron	1.4 mg	8%
Magnesium	6.8 mg	2%
Phosphorus	13.6 mg	1%
Potassium	176 mg	5%
Sodium	13.6 mg	1%
Zinc	0.7 mg	5%
Copper	0.1 mg	6%
Manganese	0.3 mg	14%
Selenium	2.7 mcg	4%
Fluoride	23.7 mcg	

Nutrition Facts

Serving Size 339 g (1 Cup)

Amount Per Serving

Calories 1031   Calories from Fat 0

	% Daily Value*
Total Fat 0g	0%
Saturated Fat 0g	0%
Trans Fat 0g	
Cholesterol 0mg	0%
Sodium 14mg	1%
Total Carbohydrate 279g	93%
Dietary Fiber 1g	3%
Sugars 278g	
Protein 1g	

Vitamin B6	4%	•	Vitamin C	3%
Riboflavin	8%	•	Folate	2%

*Percent Daily Values are based on a 2,000 calorie diet. Your daily values may be higher or lower depending on your calorie needs.

http://www.benefits-of-honey.com/honey-nutrition.html

Chapter 3
Cleansetox Do's & Don'ts

People always wonder about vitamins while on the Cleansetox or any cleansing and I wondered the same thing. I took them once because I am kind of stubborn and it made me queasy. I was thinking more is better and not so much.

Do not take vitamins while on Cleansetox it's not necessary since all your nutrients are provided as long as you are following the Cleanse correctly.

Lemons are a loosening/cleansing food with lots of important building factors. Between the lemons, limes, oranges, maple syrup and cayenne pepper working together you get amazing results like the following:

1. It's over 50% potassium helps strengthen the heart, builds the adrenal glands and kidneys.
2. It increases your oxygen which builds vitality.
3. The carbon is a motor stimulant.
4. Hydrogen helps the sensory nervous system.
5. Natural calcium helps to build lungs.
6. Phosphorus aids your bones, builds brain to lift brain fog.
7. Sodium helps with tissue building.
8. Magnesium is a blood alkalizer.
9. All the iron helps quickly correct anemia.
10. Chlorine cleans the blood plasma.
11. Silicon helps the thyroid for deeper and better breathing.

By taking in natural iron, copper, calcium, carbon and hydrogen it makes a great combination for cleansing, building and healing. Supplements may interfere with the natural cleansing process.

<u>How to Properly Break the Cleansetox Early</u>

If you have to stop the Cleanse or want to stop only after being on one or two days.

1. Sip on Orange juice throughout the first day off the Cleanse and sipping on water as well.
2. Sip on Orange juice and add vegetable soup second day. See Recipes for vegetable soup.
3. Continue with the Orange juice and vegetable soup for the third day
4. Resume your normal eating fourth day off of Cleanse.

<u>Pregnancy and Breast Feeding</u>

If you are pregnant and/or breast feeding do not go on the Cleansetox.

<u>Cravings</u>

Whatever your body is eliminating is what you will crave. These cravings will be gone with the next day's eliminations. This is good to know so that you will realize the cravings will vanish by the next day, so hang in there.

<u>Irritability</u>

On every diet and or weight loss plan I am irritable and it's a known fact most dieters are. The reason for it is because you are taking in less food and allowing your body to detox. One symptom of cleansing/detoxing is irritability. You're not alone, so hang with it I promise it will be worth it.

Bored and Anxious

Yeah you guessed it a couple more symptoms of cleansing are boredom and anxiousness. You may find yourself wanting to chew something while being bored and I would chew on a straw, the straw I use to drink my lemonade. If it helps to the finish line do it.

Aches and Pains

Everyone is different, so you may have many aches and pains, a few or none. In my experience with myself and others is if we have had any aches and pains its short lived. Usually in a couple of days it's gone. Some severe cases like heavy coffee drinkers might take 4 days, but then its smooth sailing.

Fatigue

Of course you will feel fatigued at first since toxins age you and make you tired.

Burning Bowel Movements

Since you are using cayenne pepper your bowel movements may burn. Especially for those of us that like it more spicy. I use about 3 times the amount of cayenne pepper. Another reason is toxins and waste are acidic and can cause burning.

Don't confuse Cravings with Hunger

Often times you are just dehydrated and need more water. Another way to tell you are having a craving is if you are craving Pizza and you are offered a salad and turn it down that's just a craving. Let's face it if you are truly Hungary you will scarf the salad down.

Tongue Coating

You will find you have a white coating over your tongue and that is the toxins you are releasing. Towards the end of 10 days your tongue should be clean and pink, if it's not then you are probably still detoxing out waste.

Brushing your teeth

Use a little baking soda and water. Form you a paste and brush with just baking soda and water.

Emotional Detox

It seems about day four I feel so emotionally drained and that is what others have said that I work with. It can happen at any time though, just know it's normal.

Diarrhea

If you are experiencing diarrhea that is normal, but if it goes on for four days or longer then discontinue doing the Cleanse. It's normal to have diarrhea for two to three days because of the release of so much toxic waste. If your diarrhea continues after discontinuing the Cleanse you should probably go see your doctor since diarrhea can be serious.

Exercising

It's not necessary to exercise. I recommend you walk 20 minutes daily just because it's so good for you to move and it will help move the toxic waste out faster. Walk only if you're able to and want to.

Taking it easy

You may need to take it easy if you are severely overweight, if you are on a lot of medications, if you have a lot of allergies and last but not least if you are elderly.

Colognes, Perfumes and Other

Since you are cleansing your system of toxins its best to not use colognes, perfumes, lotions and other beauty products. Unless you have natural things like using coconut oil and such. Another thing to abstain from is using cleaning products unless they are all natural like a vinegar based solution.

Chapter 4
Frequently Asked Questions

Here's a list of questions often asked and things I have wondered about before starting my cleansing.

How do I get my Protein?

First off this is blown way out of proportion since our bodies are only 16% protein. Once you realized pure protein is mostly nitrogen, oxygen and hydrogen along with some carbon. The oxygen, hydrogen and some carbon we get from the air. Nitrogen is approximately four times the amount in the same air as there is oxygen. We build and assimilate these things in our bodies as protein as well.

Is Water Fasting good?

Water fasting is fine for a day, but outside of that I would say no. You are losing too many nutrients, whereas with cleansing you are getting water and nutrients to replenish your body and mind. It's also just not necessary.

Salt Water Cleansing

If you prefer the salt water cleansing by all means go that route. I couldn't endure it and most of my clients could not either, so I promote herbal tea for bowel movement. The salt water cleansing is 32 ounces of water with 2 level teaspoons of sea salt.

How many lemons, limes and oranges should I buy?

First off make sure they are organic. I would buy for no more than 5 days at a time. About 40 lemons, 60 limes and 20 oranges is what I get. It always varies a little depending on the sizes of the fruit.

How come you allow green veggies?

Green veggies are all naturally detoxing food, so it does not stop your cleansing. Another reason is some people have a hard time making it and if they can have some green veggies and cross the finish line then go for it. It also helps when you finish the fast to assimilate food again.

Why would I go with Cleansetox over the Master Cleanse?

The Master Cleanse is great and works. The difference is the Cleansetox has more options to get the same job done. On the Cleansetox you get raw green veggies if you want, the cleanse formula has lemons, limes and oranges, so you get a better taste and you can use honey instead of maple syrup. The Master Cleanse was written in 1976 and a lot of research and studies has been done since on how veggies are naturally cleansing and about how honey has so many healing health nutrients that it appears almost endless.

What about medications?

You need to consult your physician over this. I was on thyroid, I was diabetic, high cholesterol, high blood pressure, cancer and I am healed and off all medications. I was only taking medications for thyroid and high cholesterol, but my doctor wanted me to take mediations for my other diseases and I said no. I went on several cleanses and was on a mostly raw plant based diet to cleanse my system of disease.

Remember we are all different and will all have different experiences. One thing is certain we will all feel better by cleansing the toxins out of our systems.

How much weight can I lose?

It varies how much you lose. Depends on what you weigh to begin with, what is your health condition, did you follow the Cleanse exactly as directed, what is your age, how active are you? If you are not super thin and a little over weight you will most likely lose between 15 and 20 pounds. If you are fairly overweight then you will most likely drop 20 or more pounds in ten days. Also, you will drop a lot of inches at the same time.

Beyond Cleansetox

No matter how many days you go on the Cleansetox you should incorporate 50 percent of your food intake as raw veggies and fruit to naturally help detox daily. I recommend you still do the Cleansetox every quarter, three months, or twice a year, every six months, to keep your system in great running order.

We are all different and think some of us may need meat or operate better with meat. If you are one that needs meat just make sure its Organic, clean of hormones and antibiotics. You should get away from dairy unless its raw milk because the processing of dairy removes important nutrients.

Remember to drink plenty of water and some form of movement daily even if it's just walking.

Another important thing that is so helpful is to journal. Journal causes you to focus and get in touch with your feelings and often times is like an emotional detox.

Meditation is another healing way I recommend. Meditation causes you to slow down and smell the roses so to speak. It's very healing to bond with your inner self and meditation helps with that.

Chapter 5
Recipes and Charts

Soup Recipes

Broccoli Cauliflower Soup Diet

Ingredients:

16 ounces	Broccoli Flowerets (fresh or frozen)
16 ounces	Cauliflower Flowerets (fresh or frozen)
1 large	Onion
2	Green Bell Peppers
16 ounces	Chicken Broth fat free or Vegetable Broth
1 packet	Lipton Beefy Onion Soup mix
16 ounces	Rotel Tomatoes or stewed tomatoes or tomato sauce
	Sea Salt and Pepper for taste

Instructions:

Chop all vegetables place in a 4 quart stock pot. Add chicken broth, Lipton Beefy Onion Soup mix packet and Rotel tomatoes. Add enough water to just cover the soup mixture. Stir soup mixture and turn heat on to medium low. Add Sea salt and pepper to taste. Let simmer for about 2 hours. Refrigerate leftovers.

Brussel Sprout Soup Diet

Ingredients:

16 ounces	Brussel Sprouts (fresh or frozen)
1 large	Onion
2	Bell Peppers (green, yellow, red or orange)
2 stalks	Celery
16 ounces	Chicken Broth fat free
16 ounces	Stewed Tomatoes
	Sea Salt and Pepper for taste

Instructions:

Chop all vegetables, except the **Brussel Sprouts**, place in a 4 quart stock pot. Add chicken broth and stewed tomatoes. Add enough water to just cover the soup mixture. Stir soup mixture and turn heat on to medium low. Add Sea salt and pepper to taste. Let simmer for about 2 hours. Refrigerate leftovers.

Cabbage Soup Diet

Ingredients:

1 head	Green Cabbage
1 large	Onion
2	Green Bell Peppers
2 stalks	Celery
16 ounces	Chicken Broth fat free
1 packet	Lipton Onion Soup mix
32 ounces	Stewed Tomatoes
1 tsp	Onion Powder, optional
1 tsp	Garlic Powder, optional
	Sea Salt and Pepper for taste

Instructions:

Chop all vegetables place in a 4 quart stock pot. Add chicken broth, Lipton Onion Soup mix packet and stewed tomatoes. Add enough water to just cover the soup mixture. Stir soup mixture and turn heat on to medium low. Add garlic power, onion powder, Sea salt and pepper to taste. Let simmer for about 2 hours. Refrigerate leftovers.

Green Bean Soup Diet

Ingredients:

24 ounces	Green Beans (Frozen or Fresh)
1 large	Onion
16 ounces	Chicken Broth fat free
1 packet	Lipton Savory Herb and Garlic Onion Soup Mix
16 ounces	Diced Tomatoes
	Sea Salt and Pepper for taste

Instructions:

Chop all vegetables place in a 4 quart stock pot. Add chicken broth, Lipton Savory Herb and Garlic Onion Soup mix packet and diced tomatoes. Add enough water to just cover the soup mixture. Stir soup mixture and turn heat on to medium low. Add sea salt and pepper to taste. Let simmer for about 2 hours. Refrigerate leftovers.

Snow Pea Soup Diet

Ingredients:

16 ounces	Snow Peas (fresh or frozen)
1 large	Onion
2	Yellow Bell Peppers
2 stalks	Celery
16 ounces	Chicken Broth fat free
1 packet	Lipton Onion Soup mix
16 ounces	Rotel Tomatoes
	Sea Salt and Pepper for taste

Instructions:

Chop all vegetables place in a 4 quart stock pot. Add chicken broth, Lipton Onion Soup mix packet and Rotel tomatoes. Add enough water to just cover the soup mixture. Stir soup mixture and turn heat on to medium low. Add Sea salt and pepper to taste. Let simmer for about 2 hours. Refrigerate leftovers.

Squash Soup Diet

Ingredients:

16 ounces	Yellow Squash (frozen or fresh)
16 ounces	Green Zucchini (frozen or fresh)
1 large	Onion
2	Red Bell Peppers
16 ounces	Chicken Broth fat free
1 packet	Lipton Onion Mushroom Soup mix
32 ounces	Rotel Tomatoes
	Sea Salt and Pepper for taste

Instructions:

Chop all vegetables place in a 4 quart stock pot. Add chicken broth, Lipton Onion Mushroom Soup mix packet and Rotel tomatoes. Add enough water to just cover the soup mixture. Stir soup mixture and turn heat on to medium low. Add Sea salt and pepper to taste. Let simmer for about 2 hours. Refrigerate leftovers.

Variations with the soup recipes are you can replace the Lipton soup mix with dehydrated veggie powders such as okra powder. You can replace the chicken broth with vegetable broth. Always make sure on the broth you get the organic to stay away from MSG and other toxins.

You can substitute just about any of the veggies with others. Stay away from potatoes, corn and any other high starch veggies until resuming normal eating.

Body Recipes

Body Smoother

Ingredients:

¼ cup crushed pecans
½ cup almond oil or your favorite nut oil
¼ cup coconut sugar
1 tsp vanilla extract

Directions:

Stir ingredients together, and then place into a jar with a lid. After cleansing skin in the shower, while you are still in the shower massage a small scoop of the scrub over dry, flaky areas. Rinse and pat dry. Keeps for about 4 weeks.

Breakouts be gone

Ingredients:

2 Tbs. cranberry juice – 100% juice.
½ cup of Witch Hazel

Directions:

Pour ingredients into a clean, reclose able bottle. Wash face and shake bottle, then pour some toner onto a cotton pad and wipe over your face. Keeps for up to two weeks in the refrigerator.

Ahhh Mocha Body Polish

Ingredients:

1 cup of brown sugar
½ cup olive oil or almond oil
2 Tbs. ground coffee
2 Tbs. cocoa power
4 drops peppermint essential oil

Directions:

Mix all the ingredients in a large bowl and stir well until completely mixed well. Start from your toes to your shoulders by applying a thin layer and gently rubbing the mixture into your skin using small circles then rinse well.

Ahhh Whipped Cocoa Body Butter

Ingredients:

1 cup of coconut oil
3 drops of cacao essential oil
3 drops of peppermint essential oil

Directions:

Combine all ingredients in a bowl. Use a mixer and whip mixture on high until they become fluffy and kinda airy, for five minutes. Smooth as much as needed over dry skin and store the rest in a jar. Good for three months.

Citrus Scrub

Ingredients:

1 Small dark glass jar/container 4 to 6 Oz
1 small bowl
3 oz coarse sea salt
1 oz almond oil
9 drops grapefruit essential oil
9 drops lemon essential oil
10 drops lavender essential oil
7 drops of tangerine essential oil
7 drops of orange essential oil

Directions:

Combine almond oil and all essential oils in bowl first then add coarse sea salt a little at a time stirring until you have consistency of a thick paste. Let paste sit for one hour then pour into to jar. If kept in covered and stored in dark glass container will last for six months.

Happy Feet Smoother

Ingredients:

½ cup coarse sea salt
2 oz olive oil
5 drops grapefruit essential oil
5 drops orange essential oil
6 drops lemon essential oil
6 drops lime essential oil
10 drops Rosemary essential oil
10 drops lavender essential oil
1 sprig of Rosemary leaf chopped finely (optional)

Directions:

Combine all ingredients together in a bowl and mix well then set aside. Soak feet in very warm water for 15 minutes to soften the skin. Next slather mixture on your feet and really concentrating on any rough patches. Once finished rubbing mixture on feet wrap feet I plastic wrap and wrap in warm towel. Leave feet wrapped for 20 minutes and rinse well with warm water.

Warming Bath Infusion

Ingredients:

2 Tbs. of almond oil or olive oil
4 drops of Rosemary essential oil
4 drops of basil essential oil
4 drops of sage essential oil
4 drops of Marjoram essential oil

Combine oils in a small cup and start filling bath with warm water and place cup of mixture under warm running bath water to let the mixture flow through the bath water and soak for thirty minutes. Make bath as warm as you can handle, but be careful not to get it to hot so that you

Face Brightener

Ingredients:

1 small apple, peeled, cored and grated
2 Tbs. Coconut Sugar

Directions:

Mix the ingredients together until they form a grainy paste. Massage gently over clean, damp skin with circular motions. Rinse and pat dry.

Yields 1 Treatment application

Cristie's Seaweed Body & Face Mask

This mask is great for getting rid of Cellulite, but is great for your whole body and face. Remember to always use organic and check labels for chemicals and additives.

Ingredients:
½ cup Green Clay
½ cup Seaweed
¼ cup fresh lime juice
1 tbsp honey
3 tbsp hot water
5 drops of Grapefruit Oil

Directions:
Grind up the seaweed and add to green clay. Mix in the lime juice, honey, hot water and Grapefruit oil. Coat your areas you tend to treat and wrap with plastic for 25 minutes and of course you don't wrap your face. After wrapped with plastic for 25 minutes rinse off in the shower. I use twice a week.
Coat your face and lie down in a comfortable are and just lay really warm wet cloth on face for 25 minutes. Do not press wet cloth into face just lightly lay on your face. Make sure you can breathe at all times.
If you don't like Grapefruit oil then replace the Grapefruit oil with another essential oil like Jasmine.
Happy Wrapping to pure beauty!

Pumpkin Pore Shrinking Mask

Ingredients:

2 Tbs fresh Pumpkin
1 Tbs. Plain Greek Yogurt
1 Tbs. Honey

Directions:

Mix all the ingredients together until creamy. Wash and dry face, smooth the mask on your face. Relax and let sit 20 minutes. Rinse and pat dry.

Yields 1 Treatment Mask

Salt Skin Softening Scrub

Ingredients:

1 Cup sea salt (preferably Celtic, Himalayan pink salt or Hawaiian red salt)
1 cup Olive or Almond Oil

Directions:

Combine ingredients and mix well. Gently run onto your skin in circular motions before shower. To avoid any mess put on your skin in the shower then turn the shower on and rinse off. Pat dry and follow with a moisturizer.

Cookie Body Scrub

Ingredients:

2 Cups of brown sugar
1 cup of almond oil
2 tsp vanilla
6 to 7 drops of essential oil ginger

Directions:

Combine and mix all the ingredients in a bowl with a wooden spoon. Put in an air tight seal container that is BPA free. It's good for one month. Be sure to put date on label on container. When you take a shower just massage in a circular motion starting with your feet and work your way up your whole body. This will help flush out all those toxins out of your system. Be sure to rinse your body well and pat dry. Enjoy!

Cookie Facial Masque

Ingredients:

½ cup of water
4 to 5 drops of ginger essential oil
3 Tbs of oatmeal (not the minute oatmeal)
1 tsp of Honey or Grade B Maple Syrup
½ cup of canned Coconut Cream

Directions:

Bring water to a boil and quickly remove pan from heat, add oatmeal and soak for 5 minutes. Strain out the oatmeal and all the remaining ingredients except the essential oil. Mix well and place in freezer for 10 to 15 minutes or until cool and firm. Add essential oil and mix. Use fingertips to apply over your clean face and neck, but avoid the eye area. Leave on for 20 minutes, rinse and pat dry.

Relaxing cookie bath

Ingredients:

1 cup of Almond oil
5 to 6 drops of Ginger essential oil
1 cup of baking soda
1 cup brown sugar
1 cup of Epson salt

Directions:

Place all ingredients in a blender and blend until smooth. Pour into cookie mold pan, refrigerate overnight and store in air tight container. When you're ready take a cookie and put in a nice hot bath. Light some candles and enjoy.

Cleansetox Chart

1 cup laxative tea morning or evening	32 ounces Cleansetox Morning Drink	32 Ounces Cleansetox Noon Drink	32 Ounces Cleansetox Evening Drink	Comments/Feelings/Ideas
Day 1				
Day 2				
Day 3				
Day 4				
Day 5				
Day 6				
Day 7				
Day 8				
Day 9				
Day 10				
Day 11				
Day 12				
Day 13				
Day 14				
Day 15				
Day 16				
Day 17				

Cleansetox Chart

1 cup laxative tea morning or evening	32 ounces Cleansetox Morning Drink	32 Ounces Cleansetox Noon Drink	32 Ounces Cleansetox Evening Drink	Comments/Feelings/Ideas
Day 1				
Day 2				
Day 3				
Day 4				
Day 5				
Day 6				
Day 7				
Day 8				
Day 9				
Day 10				
Day 11				
Day 12				
Day 13				
Day 14				
Day 15				
Day 16				
Day 17				

Cleansetox Chart

1 cup laxative tea morning or evening	32 ounces Cleansetox Morning Drink	32 Ounces Cleansetox Noon Drink	32 Ounces Cleansetox Evening Drink	Comments/Feelings/Ideas
Day 1				
Day 2				
Day 3				
Day 4				
Day 5				
Day 6				
Day 7				
Day 8				
Day 9				
Day 10				
Day 11				
Day 12				
Day 13				
Day 14				
Day 15				
Day 16				
Day 17				

Cleansetox Chart

1 cup laxative tea morning or evening	32 ounces Cleansetox Morning Drink	32 Ounces Cleansetox Noon Drink	32 Ounces Cleansetox Evening Drink	Comments/Feelings/Ideas
Day 1				
Day 2				
Day 3				
Day 4				
Day 5				
Day 6				
Day 7				
Day 8				
Day 9				
Day 10				
Day 11				
Day 12				
Day 13				
Day 14				
Day 15				
Day 16				
Day 17				

Cleansetox Chart

1 cup laxative tea morning or evening	32 ounces Cleansetox Morning Drink	32 Ounces Cleansetox Noon Drink	32 Ounces Cleansetox Evening Drink	Comments/Feelings/Ideas
Day 1				
Day 2				
Day 3				
Day 4				
Day 5				
Day 6				
Day 7				
Day 8				
Day 9				
Day 10				
Day 11				
Day 12				
Day 13				
Day 14				
Day 15				
Day 16				
Day 17				

Date Started: _____ Weight:_____

Measurements: Chest_____ Waist:_____ Hips:_____ Thighs:_____

Overall
Feelings:_____
_____
_____
_____
_____
_____
_____
_____
_____
_____
_____
_____
_____

Date Finished:_____ Weight:_____

Measurements: Chest_____ Waist:_____ Hips:_____ Thighs:_____

Overall
Feelings:_____
_____
_____
_____
_____
_____
_____
_____
_____
_____
_____

Date Started: _____ Weight:_____

Measurements: Chest_____ Waist:_____ Hips:_____ Thighs:_____

Overall
Feelings:_____
_____
_____
_____
_____
_____
_____
_____
_____
_____
_____
_____
_____

Date Finished:_____ Weight:_____

Measurements: Chest_____ Waist:_____ Hips:_____ Thighs:_____

Overall
Feelings:_____
_____
_____
_____
_____
_____
_____
_____
_____
_____
_____
_____

Date Started: _____ Weight:_____

Measurements: Chest_____ Waist:_____ Hips:_____ Thighs:_____

Overall
Feelings:_____
_____
_____
_____
_____
_____
_____
_____
_____
_____
_____
_____

Date Finished:_____ Weight:_____

Measurements: Chest_____ Waist:_____ Hips:_____ Thighs:_____

Overall
Feelings:_____
_____
_____
_____
_____
_____
_____
_____
_____
_____
_____

Date Started: _____ Weight:_____

Measurements: Chest_____ Waist:_____ Hips:_____ Thighs:_____

Overall
Feelings:_____
_____
_____
_____
_____
_____
_____
_____
_____
_____
_____
_____

Date Finished:_____ Weight:_____

Measurements: Chest_____ Waist:_____ Hips:_____ Thighs:_____

Overall
Feelings:_____
_____
_____
_____
_____
_____
_____
_____
_____
_____
_____

Date Started: _____ Weight:_____

Measurements: Chest_____ Waist:_____ Hips:_____ Thighs:_____

Overall
Feelings:_____
_____
_____
_____
_____
_____
_____
_____
_____
_____
_____
_____

Date Finished:_____ Weight:_____

Measurements: Chest_____ Waist:_____ Hips:_____ Thighs:_____

Overall
Feelings:_____
_____
_____
_____
_____
_____
_____
_____
_____
_____
_____

Chapter 6
Recommended Readings & Links

Links:

www.cbwill.com

www.healthtidings.com

http://www.integrativenutrition.com/

http://www.benefits-of-honey.com/

http://www.whfoods.com/index.php

http://www.mercola.com/

http://www.greenmedinfo.com/

Reading:

Books by Cristie Will
http://www.amazon.com/-
/e/B00VW32UZM?ref_=pe_1724030_132998070

Books by Linda Yalen
Last One Standing

Books by Pam Grout

Books by Mark Hyman

Books by David Wolfe

Conclusion

My hope is to help as many people as I can to gain their health back and lose some weight along the way.

I have provided you with the fastest, healthiest and better tasking way to cleanse, lose weight and gain energy to a vibrancy you haven't felt in years.

We don't have to have the massive ill health that seems to be plaguing us today. From all the fast foods, processed foods, toxins in the air we breathe, beauty skin care products, cleaning products, lawn and garden products it's no wonder we are sick.

I encourage you to cleanse two to 4 times a year along with incorporating a healthy diet.

I would love to hear from you about your Cleansetox cleanse. Please email me at healthtidings@outlook.com.

Here's to your new Vibrant Health!

Cristie

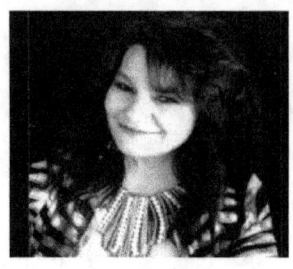

Cristie Will, BBA, CHC, CIC
Author

Cristie was born and raised in Hobbs, New Mexico. She moved to Colorado 18 years ago and still living there loving all the beauty Colorado has to offer. She has a daughter Lauren and a son Josh along with beautiful grandchildren. She has been an accountant the last 30 years. Not only an accountant and Health Coach but a teacher as well, teaching QuickBooks, cooking, detoxing and weight loss classes too!

In 2012, she lost her husband to lung cancer. After losing her husband to lung cancer she needed to make changes in her own health, so she did. Cristie went through a life transformation losing 200 pounds and went back to school to become a Nutritional Heath Coach adding Cleansing Intensive certification. She obtained her education from Institute of Integrative Nutrition for her Health Coaching. Her education for the Cleansing Intensive education was under Dr. Terry Willard CIH, PHD at the Wild Rose College. She is currently studying to add FDN, Functional Diagnostic Nutritionist to her skills to be able to help even more people.

Besides helping others, Cristie's other passion is to write. She has written 5 cookbooks, 2 of them are political collector's cookbooks. She didn't stop with cookbooks she also wrote "Veteran's Day Chase, a CIA political thriller, along with a QuickBooks Step by Step Guide. She has written 4 health and weight loss books. Last but not least she published a Car buying guide that her late husband had written with his vast knowledge and experience in the car industry.

NOTES

NOTES

NOTES

NOTES

NOTES

www.ingramcontent.com/pod-product-compliance
Lightning Source LLC
Chambersburg PA
CBHW070820290526
45795CB00002B/779